Ph

Super Nu

MW01285366

By
James Paul

* * * * *

PUBLISHED BY:
James Paul

Phytonutrients: Super Nutrient Powerhouses

Table of Contents

Introduction

We've been told for generations to eat our fruits and vegetables, because they are good for us. What we normally aren't told as children however is how items in our body such as DNA for example are hurt, free radicals damage our bodies, etc. We're also not told how good for us plants and fruit actually are, including on the labels of the food we buy.

Part of the reason that labels do not include what their nutritional properties do, is because of potential litigation. We all know the benefits of protein, in that it aids in muscle maintenance as well as calcium which helps us build strong bones. We've been told for years that fish is brain food, but rarely will you ever see a label saying that the blueberry compound it contains could fight cancer!

Any conspiracy theorist will tell you the reason the true and amazing powers of plants (particularly fruits and vegetables) is because the pharmaceutical industry will lose too much money. That could be true, however this sentence contains a keyword that also relates to why the previous statement is a theory. Science is based on facts, not "could be" situations.

Having many years as a sales agent for a nutritional chain, I have heard and seen my share of stories relating to the power behind phytonutrients. I have seen proof that there is some massive power behind these phytonutrients, and I have also seen them taken for conditions they are "known" for and have no effect.

I will say, personally I prefer the natural route which led to me studying a variety of nutrients and their potential biochemical reactions. I, myself and only speaking for myself, am sold hard on the fact they work. Do they work for everyone? I have never seen that.

With that being said, I need to cover myself, and would appreciate you read this small disclaimer. I am not, nor was I ever, licensed to practice medicine of any form. I can tell you unless the requirements change dramatically I never will be as I have no desire to go back to school for it. I will say I am overly wise, and am a lifelong student in that I read regularly and am very - very - good at fact checking evidence and information.

Whatever you read in this book, may or may not be approved by your doctor. He may not agree with anything I say, which is fine as this isn't a mandatory field doctors have to study. Whatever route you decide to go, you need to realize this book is for informational and educational purposes only. I cannot and will not make any effort to encourage you to cease any treatment now or in the future encouraged by your doctor. I will never claim anything in here to be "medical advice" as I am not a doctor. You accept that anything you take away from this book is your decision and you will be wise enough to inform your doctor.

Back to the interesting stuff, you will learn a lot about phytonutrients in this book (some call them phytochemicals, I'll get into that also!) I'll let you know what I learn about everything phyto. You'll gain some insight into the major classes of phytonutrients and you will learn a ton about what they are believed to do. That last part is the biggest reason I have been studying them for ages.

The book will contain a bunch of sarcasm, my own weird twist on things, as well as a humorous take on whatever I can. There's a reason for that, and I'll even tell you why (the sarcasm begins). Unless you are a (cool) geek like me, the idea of science is extremely dull and boring. I never did well with science in school (okay, I did, but English and sociology were better grade-wise and business classes received the bulk of my interest) because my teachers could not make it interesting. This is a topic which is near and dear to my passion, health, and something I really believe you should know. I won't get into the rants I am famous for (I know that because I wrote this part last.

Although I may joke around occasionally and potentially even throw in a footnote, the subject matter behind the jokes is far more serious. It is my way of getting you to stay with me and truly gain an understanding for a very under discussed topic, which I believe we will only break the tip of the iceberg on in our lifetime. This is also one of the longest paragraphs in this book, mainly consisting of a ramble with a purpose and not a rant.

Dedication

The idea of nutrition is something that means a lot to me, and is a concept I feel should be shared with the world. The mission of this book is to provide my findings, although not medical advice, in the hopes these wonders of phytonutrients begin receiving a lot more credit.

I truly believe in the idea that God gave us the fruits and plants we need to sustain life, a vibrant and healthy life, far past the age of 100. Possible or not is non-fundamental, it is the faith behind the concept that keeps the faith instilled in me since birth burning.

This book, I am hoping motivates individuals to gain a passion into the curious and powerful world of phytonutrients. I do believe the cure for almost every world health condition lays in one phytonutrient. Although there are far too many for one page, which is where the rest of this book comes in, I do believe they each have a health healing purpose.

Who this book is for......

My children, I truly hope you eat your fruits and vegetables, and remain vibrant far past my times. The illnesses and conditions that had struck me early in life, although are near non-existent or are gone completely, are things I would not in my worst nightmare dream of you dealing with. Or you children (I don't want to be a grandfather before I am 60, just saying).

My selfish desires, my grandmother was taken far too early from me and caused emotional grief I wouldn't wish bestowed upon anyone outside of the fiery bowels of Hell. I want that prevented. My niece Aubrie, I pray someone can find something to give these ideas and research scientific proof and rid you of Cystic Fibrosis.

For the malnourished, sickly, and overly vaccinated children and adults of the world. I really do wish we could all be happy, healthy, wealthy, and wise. This book won't make you a millionaire, nor myself (unless God grants me an awesome blessing) but I also believe we are what we eat.

For you reading this, I hope this gives you the desire to take your health more seriously and maybe, just maybe, prevent or help ward off genetical issue that inflict fear and torment in your family.

The Shortest Chapter : Phytonutrient Versus Phytochemical

So what is the difference between phytos in regards to nutrients and chemicals? Easy, some people are picky and call the nutrients chemicals because of the activities they do! Told you this was going to be a short chapter, we're all done!

Many phytonutrients, especially flavonoids, are considered to be a secondary plant metabolite. What's a secondary metabolite? What's a primary plant metabolite? WHAT'S A PLANT METABOLITE?! We're going to cover those questions, and there's an important aspect to this part. We're going to start understanding, before we get into phytonutrients, how these metabolites play a pivotal role in plants and act eerily similar in us, humans (unless this is being read in the year 3500 A.D. and primates can read and have some form of legal humanistic protection, than I apologize - using the word humans wasn't politically correct)..

What's a plant secondary metabolite? Let's see!

Being considered a plant secondary metabolite means that, well let's look at a hockey term. When you have the second string in during hockey, they come in to help protect the team, a goalie could also be seen as a plant secondary metabolite. You won't win a game with zero goals, right? In fact sometimes to score that goal the first string is on the rink with another player and the goalie is completely removed. But what do the second string and goalie actually do then? They protect the offence from having to work harder. The defense attacks the other side's offense when the mid point line is penetrated, and they protect the goalie.

Like a hockey game, plant secondary metabolites are crucial, but not imperative to a team's chances at winning. Following me so far? Plant secondary metabolites are the plant's second string, they actually facilitate the primary functions of the plant! The secondary metabolites keep the plants systems working properly.

The secondary metabolites do things like fighting off herbivores (plant eating species), they scare away pests, and they also defend against pathogens by putting them in full Nelson's and making the pathogen scream uncle! The last part is a bit of a stretch, pathogens can't scream nor can a secondary metabolite trap anything in a full Nelson. But if they could they would.

It's not just giving out Nelson's or fighting pathogens away that make the secondary plant metabolites so crucial to their life. They are also plant hormones, the hormones deal with the regulation of the important area of metabolic activity and sort of act as a supervisor by watching over the plant's development.

Want to look into primary metabolites and secondary metabolites a little deeper? Great, I was going to anyway especially since it will allow you to see a correlation between how the primary and secondary metabolites in plants act similarly in us. The easiest way to see the difference in primary and secondary metabolites are is with their name usage.

Primary metabolites are obviously the most important. They promote and produce what is needed for the plant's survival. Instead of going through a hockey analogy again as baseball is by far my favorite sports (could have used it earlier, couldn't I) we'll look at ourselves.

What do we need to survive naturally? We need our heart, lungs, and brain to be fully functional, right? Those are our primary metabolites (even though we aren't synthesizing them and they come pre installed). Our secondary metabolite is an immune system for ease of sake. If our brain isn't working, we are medically dead, right? If we don't have an immune system, are we dead? No, the immune system plays the pinnacle role in us as the defense mechanisms play in the plant. We can survive without a working immune system, we just get much sicker. Everything is starting to make more sense now, right? We know that certain synthesized metabolites help the plant stay healthy and fight off disease and pathogens. Have you ever heard of garlic fighting off mosquitoes? How about blueberries potentially warding off cancer? Seeing how those secondary plant metabolites work in us?

Metabolites also help to dictate which color a plant is going to be, why's that important? Different colors will attract different pollinators to help the sex cycle (growth, seeding, etc - I figured using sex cycle would wake you up if you're nodding off).

What On Earth Is A Phytonutrient?

The simplest explanation I can give you toward what a phytonutrient is, is that it is a noun. The explanation beyond that is slightly more confusing. Phytonutrient is derived from the Greek word phyto, which means plant. A nutrient is a source of nourishment, mainly an ingredient in food, considering the base word it's a compound as plants (grown naturally) do not have ingredients. That's it. If we put the words together we have planned (I'll throw the word based in here as it fits well) nourishment. Now if you are ever asked what I phytonutrient is at a dinner party or graduation event you can tell the person asking that a phytonutrient is a plant compound. Doing so will probably make them assume you are brilliant.

Are you assuming that we need phytonutrients to live? If you answered yes, you are on the same page as I am and scientifically incorrect! Are you now asking yourself "really?!", yes phytonutrients are widely considered non-essential nutrients. How does that make sense? Let's take a peak.

Phytonutrients are extremely important, and in many cases have shown amazing and extremely powerful health properties. The reason that these are non-essential is that they are not solely responsible for us staying alive, maintaining metabolism, or functioning. That job ultimately falls into the hands of essential nutrients such as minerals, vitamins, fats, carbohydrates, and proteins. Still confused? I have an unrelated in nature, but very related in principle, example below to help you out.

To better grasp the concept of non-essential versus essential nutrients let's look at my favorite topic aside from health and business (unless you consider PED's and money), which is baseball. For a baseball team to be eligible to play during the regular season you must be able to have a 25 man roster. You need 3 outfielders as well as 4 infielders along with a pitcher and catcher.

The above example would be our essential nutrients, this part is where we start to really understand the non-essential aspect of nutrients. Getting back to baseball, that basic team would not win the World Series when adding in the fact of All Stars and future Hall of Fame players (which unfortunately my 2013 Blue Jay's have none of). This is where our phytonutrient baseball players come in. We have specialty men (right handed, left handed, and other situational pitchers), pinch runners, pinch hitters, and so on. The importance of statistics here is paramount if you want your team to have a great makeup. Too much of one will sink you in other areas whereas a balance of the additional players will make your team far better.

Did the above two examples surrounding baseball teams make this whole process easier to understand? I really hope you said yes as it's going to be tough for me to get another example. Let's look at non-nutritional life for another example.

We need air, food, and hydration (preferably water) to survive. That would be our essential nutrients. Your life would also suck pretty bad.

Non-essential items such as a car, a gorgeous wife (I have a gorgeous fiance, big improvement in my life!), a house, a table, potentially lots of money, etc. Those items would help contribute to having a better life, more fortunate if you would. Missing them unless you are obsessed with reality TV will not kill you as it would probably my youngest son's mother. This ends our examples to show the correlation and difference between nonessential and essential nutrients. If you still have doubt or uncertainty and need further explanation you are that kid in school who always raised your hand when the teacher was about to let us leave early. I'm a nice teacher though, contact me and I'll be happy to explain it more alright?

Are All Phytonutrients The Same?

Asking if all phytonutrients are the same is like saying all amino acids or vitamins do the same thing. Not all phytonutrients do the same job, and to be honest with the amount of different phytonutrients - in the thousands - it would be safe to assume they all do different things. Wondering how we can tell the differences in their properties or abilities? It's in the classes!

The differences in the classes are drastic and give more of a reason to eat a variety of fruits, vegetables, and even herbs! There are 9 widely accepted and important classes of phytonutrients. Obviously they have different properties and benefits, and I'll cover them in the following pages, it's your lucky day isn't it?

We could be hear for years, literally if this was in a different media like audio, if we went over what each and every phytonutrient property was. The classes each have a health related area they lean to. To make that part more understandable you could go back to the baseball example where you have the specialists, or even take a look at doctors. All doctors know how to do basic medical work, however if you have severe and ongoing allergy problems you'd see an Ear, Nose, and Throat, doctor or an allergist right? Let's take a quick peek at the list of phytonutrient classes (mind you these are just the most popular):

1. Carotenoids
2. Flavonoids
3. Inositol Phosphates
4. Lignans
5. Isothiocyanates
6. Phenols
7. Saponins
8. Sulfides
9. Terpenes

We're going to touch on two of these in this book, some phytonutrients have more information than other phytonutrients, and there's a very good reason for that. We know a lot more about certain phytonutrients than we do others, which is why I really hope someone reading this is motivated to research more about these natural super heros! Let's get into some details, shall we? The two we're going to focus on are believed to be the most powerful of the phytonutrients, although all are powerful and important, are the "Noids", just like the cover said!

Carotenoids: The A List

The first phytonutrient we're going to look at is the first one we listed in the bullet points, carotenoids! The reason this one comes first, is because we know the most about it. Did you know that this phytonutrient is responsible for sucking in blue light!? The result of this is deep colored, bright fruit and vegetables. Do you know what you're eating when you take in high levels of carotenoids? You're in essence eating colors, seriously. But these aren't just any colors or pigments, they are super powered as we'll discover soon (as in the next few paragraphs).

The colors synthesized by plants that are more than likely (actually, they do) are going to come in red's, oranges, and yellow's. As I mentioned, there are "branches" (no plant pun intended) of each major phytonutrient class. There are over 600 different carotenoid branches, or in other words there are more than 600 different carotenoids. The main one's are alpha-carotene, beta-carotene, beta-cryptoxanthin, lutein, lycopene, and zeaxanthin.

As if we couldn't tell by the difference in names, an approach I'll call "Not All Carotenoids Are The Same", not all carotenoids do the same thing. The most common misconception regarding carotenoids is that they are all Vitamin A, or in scientific terms provitamin A. Only a few of the main carotenoids we touched upon are provitamin A, with the pro side consisting of alpha-carotene, beta-carotene, and beta-cryptoxanthin.

What does provitamin A mean to us anyway before we decide if we should even worry about taking the other major carotenoids? Being provitamin A in regards to our body and diet means we can turn those specific carotenoids into vitamin A in our body. To be exact, we turn the provitamin A carotenoids into a by-product known as Retinol.

With all that being said it seems like we're putting down lutein,zeaxanthin, and lycopene right? The names are different (for example, they don't have a carotene type of surname [last name to us USA residents]), or any Greek effect at all (alpha and beta). So why would they be a major class of they aren't that important? If you assumed from the get go they were important, great! Actually, even though they don't produce vitamin A and pretty much have no vitamin A activity they are highly beneficial to have in your diet!

Men have a justified fear of prostate cancer, it's a man killer plain and simple. Lycopene has shown in some studies to help alleviate and decrease the effects and formation of prostate cancer, if you ask me (not just because I'm a guy) that would be pretty important in my books!

Another benefit of the "left over" carotenoids would be the fact you are able to read this, lutein as well as zeaxanthin are the only carotenoids found in our lens and retina. What are those? They're parts of your eye! It has shown in a couple epidemiological studies that the results suggest that a diet "rich" (meaning only having an abundant amount, in layer-layman words it means you have a lot of) could slow down the occurrence and development of age-related macular degeneration.

More Carotenoids - Big European Advancement Being Discussed!

There's one huge development and benefit that has been discussed greatly in Europe (we're not that far ahead in the states yet) that diets rich in the provitamin A producing carotenoids could actually help prevent and drastically slow the growth of lung cancer! If you're a heavy smoker like me, a dietary supplement of something like beta-carotene may be one of the worst things you can do.

Are you asking "why" yet? It's because in smokers the anticancer effect is actually reversed where the provitamin A carotenoids could actually increase our chances or the development of lung cancer. Talk about a hell of a reason to quit right?

If you're not a fruit and vegetable eater, I was with one 100% I especially hated eating raw vegetables. Here's the great news for us (if you're like me at least), the carotenoids are released from the source when they are lightly cooked, it tends to break anything down a bit. Obviously we're not going to overcook them. You will get some bioavailability from cutting and pureeing them as again they are being broken down.

On A Fat Free Diet? You Aren't Getting Your Carotenoid Fix!

One thing to be taken into consideration, is that although we are ingesting and digesting the food from which they come from there is no guarantee that our bodies will take in the phytonutrient intestinally. There's a bit of a magic trick around this (okay, just a way to increase the chances) and that is to take the food and have some good fats in it.

If the carotenoids aren't incorporated into a mixed micelles (which is a fancy way of saying a mixture of lipids as well as bile salts) our bodies will not absorb the carotenoids. Bummer isn't it? Let's jump back to the previous paragraph where I mentioned you should have a tiny bit of fat to absorb these nutrients. You don't need a huge tub of lard (besides, that's not a good fat) but can get away with only 3-5 grams. If you are a vain individual, don't worry this won't take away from your figure!

Flavonoids Are Phytonutrient Powerhouses!

Flavonoids are the second phytonutrient we're going to cover, and if you ask me are the most confusing. Similarly to the previously discussed carotenoids, these guys (or girls to be politically correct) are considered in a sense to be plant pigments. Let's take that one step further, and this isn't going to take away form their importance, flavonoids are also considered secondary metabolites. We know these secondary metabolites are important because we already discussed why they are before going over a phytonutrient. Right??

Want to know how large these are, these being the flavonoid class of phytonutrients? The number is believed to be around 6,000 different forms and substances. Almost every plant has a form of flavonoid to them, and there's a lot of different plants! Flavonoids provide so many different benefits at one point they were even classified as being vitamin P.

Just like carotenoids, flavonoids come in a variety of flavors (a play on the name, I would assume they're tasteless personally) and fulfill different roles. The most known role they fill is that of providing antioxidants to us, and there's a ton of different types of antioxidants provided (resveratrol, quercetin, etc.). Just to be fair, seeing I gave you a listing of the types of carotenoids, I'll do the same for flavonoids (you're welcome). But first let me explain something, aside from having similar names these phytonutrients are mainly differentiated into their groups by their chemical structure. The types of flavonoids off the flavonoid name are flavonols, flavones, flavanones, isoflavones, catechins, anthocyanidins, as well as chalcones.

Let's Talk Flavonoid Structure!

Does this sound entertaining? I didn't think so, but it is a bit interesting and I'm teaching you the in's and out's of phytonutrients so let's (briefly) cover it! I'll warn you now, this topic if you are not into science (like me) is really confusing, so I won't go crazy on it.

The structure of flavonoids is what gives them their abilities to seek out free radicals and such. At the end of the book I will give a small set of pictures relating to the structure of flavonoids.

Flavonols, Flavones, and Flavanones - What's The Difference?

If you're like me the first time you look at these three flavonoids you'd assume it's a sort of game where we're just guessing which one is spelled properly. They are similar, and at the same time different. Are you wondering if I could be anymore vague? The answer would be no, no I cannot be more vague. So let's start looking into what makes each of these different (they really are different, I promise).

Flavonols are specially structured to have a 3-hydroxyflavone backbone (the structure). What I have read and researched about this specific flavonoid is that it really protects against the oxidative stress placed on the vascular system.

Flavones have a different huge chemical/scientific make up and it appears very different to that of the flavonol. These guys have a 2-phenyl chromen-4-1 backbone. Like other flavonoids these are found primarily in fruits, vegetables, and so on right? In all actuality and this is something I found interesting regarding the flavonoid bioavailability and reach is that they are actually more plentiful in cereal as well as herbs. I literally sat and scratched my head. Flavus means yellow, right? That would be a massive depiction of where this flavonoid should come from - science proved the old language wrong apparently!

I have found the least information regarding flavanones, especially the scientific makeup and backbone which appeared to have a very minute difference between these health players and flavones. Although there's a small bit of useful information, I have found that this particular flavonoid is also one of the biggest subcategories! I found it particularly interesting that flavanone containing herbs and fruits have been used as far back as ancient China for things such as spasms and fever.

Additionally, their range of believed benefits have gone on to include help with cardiovascular issues as well as some cancers! Is that the end? No, the reach of health benefits actually extend into the bone health, cholesterol lowering, and neurodegenerative disease arenas. This is one busy flavonoid derivative!

So What's Up With Isoflavones?

These flavonoid relatives (this should have been used as a way to explain them earlier, think about family structure and you'll agree it would've been 10 times easier) can cause some confusion. When working at a vitamin chain (I left under bad terms, I won't diss - I mean drop - their name) I heard two terms interchanged with customers not blinking. Isoflavonoids and isoflavones are not the same thing! When I heard people asking for soy isoflavonoids my head would spin, but I didn't because I wanted my job at the time and it's easy to understand the confusion.

Our flavonoids so far have "family members" breaking off of the so far, right? And each of these family members have their own offspring (compounds), and the isoflavonoid is no different. The isoflavonoid is a compound inside of plants that help to give them their colors (no way! Sort of like the other phytonutrients we've hit on).

Isoflavones are much better known, as far as their popularity, as are the researched health findings. So what's an isoflavone? An isoflavone is a class of organic compounds and are related to isoflavonoids.

One very interesting aspect of isoflavones I have found is their ability to act as agonists as well as antagonists in their interaction with estrogen receptors (a major female sex hormone). They can actually mimic estrogen, and they have a really cool name as well! They're plant based naturally (isoflavones) and they deal with estrogen, any idea what they're called? Yeah, they're phytoestrogens!

Are Isoflavonoids and Isoflavones Beneficial, and What About Eating Them During Fermentation?

I'll tackle the last part first. There was reason to believe a hypothesis that stated the absorption of soy was most beneficial when you ate it in a fermented state, a la tofu. The idea was appealed in a non-scientific sense (I read legal case studies for fun too) and the idea was found to have insufficient evidence.

It is thought that isoflavonoids as well as isoflavones both have extreme health benefits, while there were some fears of adverse reactions as well. A major fear was how the phytoestrogen would work while someone was in a controlled state as far as breast cancer treatment was concerned. The fear was extremely justified especially in the beginning stages of our uncovering of all this fantastic study based findings into the Iso's (I named them that, I'm referring to both of them).

Are Soy Isoflavones Just For Women?

You may assume that, after all the phytoestrogens exhibiting estrogen like activities would in theory increase estrogen in males, right? Well, don't forget that males already have some estrogen. Would more estrogen cause man boobs though? Not really, and in fact in animal populations consuming a soy based protein diet there was evidence showing less prostate issues in regards to cancer!

Ever Heard of a Catechin? I Bet You Have (in a different name)

Catechin based supplements were one of the hottest selling products at the vitamin chain I mentioned I worked at. Many people would buy a year supply in one purchase and swore they aided them dramatically in weight loss.

Catechins are a compound related to (wait for it) flavonoids (did you see that one coming?), and are extremely popular in green tea. These are the compounds that give green tea it's main health benefits, but catechins aren't just in green tea! They're also in some foods such as cocoa (smiling ladies?) as well as cherries.

Something you should find interesting about the green tea and fat oxidation or weight loss cries is that there is extremely little evidence supporting the claims. I certainly wouldn't knock catechins and say they don't help at all with weight loss, as I believe I have seen the results based on former customer feedback (plus it's easy to tell when someone has dropped 10 pounds).

Although fat oxidation and weight loss aren't seemingly having much luck at getting the all decisive "yes it works" vote from the scientific community, there's more. If you've noticed, phytonutrients don't typically have one set job - right? A massive benefit to catechin consumption I have been following is the ridiculously high potential antioxidant activities.

Numerous studies have almost pinpointed the use and a diet consisting of consumption of catechin containing foods has shown a few things. Lower risk of serious illness, lower cardiovascular problems, lower overall mortality. I found that to be very interesting, and I personally feel much more important than preventing what we call potbelly syndrome in my area.

Although the American Heart Association and the American Cancer Association won't come out and say drink red wine and cut down on your potential for cancer and heart problems, are they really saying not to drink it? I apologize for the extra long sentence preceding this apology. Actually, the A.C.A. sort of does when it recommends limiting your intake of red wine. Am I going to give you a list of catechin containing foods? Yes I am, later on with the rest of the phytonutrients as well as some great recipes and meal plans!

Have You Had Any Anthocyanins Today?

The first time I heard this flavonoid mentioned my first thought was chemical attack by some terrorist organization. I can tell you why, I heard it for the first time shortly after the attacks in the US and due to a severe hangover I misheard the word.

This particular flavonoid is going to make your eyes open, which I hope they still are. One thing we've seen as being constant with phytonutrients is that they've all been yellow or yellowish so far, right? We can atleast say they all have yellowish crystallized structure even if they are from something yellow (I learned pea's were green in kindergarten - we'll hit a few foods with some recipes later).

Anthocyanins are from a completely different colored food! Actually, they're from a food we've hardly seen being mentioned, they're reddish to bluish colored pigments. At Least the pigments are remaining the same, right? So let's hit off some anthocyanin discussion.

Although these are the most noticeable, and have been used the longest (bilberry and elderberry) in folk medicines, the pigments from this flavonoid family member are finally getting some credit. Pharmacological (pharmaceutical) studies are even being forced to accept their use and health benefits. This is very interesting as many times things in this arena of discussion have very conclusive evidence.

I just mentioned things such as phytonutrients have inconclusive information relating to their benefits and health properties. One thing that is interesting about anthocyanins is that they are yielding the most notable evidence as being super food and highly potent antioxidants. Another very interesting thing is that science has very little idea why.

In science, especially in regards to molecules and structures, they try and peel layers away to see why something works the way it does. When it comes to anthocyanins, science isn't exactly sure if they work alone, or act as a WWE tag team idea, where one substance helps the other substance. For example, back when we talked carotenoids we mentioned how you need to take them in with some fat to be intestinally absorbed right? Same type of thinking here (although we don't need to consume fat with these guys/gals).

Unlike a few others, these pigments work on a water-soluble level. If you know anything about water-fat soluble vitamins (IE our discussion about vitamin A previously) you'll know water soluble doesn't need fat to be intestinally absorbed. Actually, I never mentioned that but now you know and knowing is half the battle, right?

Anthocyanins also prove to be very good hiders and sleepers. It appears they wait until they are triggered to start attacking the effects of stress. When they are metabolised, they also break down extremely fast making it difficult for scientists to track what they do once metabolised, aside from breaking down and hiding as I just mentioned.

Interesting So Far, Let's Talk Health Properties

You got it, what makes these flavonoids so healthy? Anthocyanins have shown to be effective against the effects and may actually protect against visual acuity harm, ARND (age-related neurodegenerative disorders), heart disease, and (not some but many) cancers.

Anthocyanins act similarly to the other flavonoid family members, they're scavengers and protectors. They are the parts of society that go out of their way to destroy and suffocate harmful free radicals from causing oxidative stress related damage.

Chalcones, Pretty Interesting Name Don't You Think?

It's a really cool name, say it with an accent and it sounds even cooler. The coolest fact about this is that it shows the true meaning of secondary plant metabolites! We've seen that many of the flavonoids, actually the other flavonoids, so far have been heavy hitters in attacking free radicals right? Consider chalcones to be similar to an advanced cavalry or special forces, they don't just hit oxidative stressors and their effects. We're going to throw antibacterial, (potentially) antiviral, antifungal, anti depressant, and anti-inflammatory powers. Sit back and say wow!

You may think that the ARND we mentioned earlier are depression based, they're not. The ARNDs I was speaking about were more along the lines of Parkinson's and Alzheimer's disease. Those conditions are believed to be caused by oxidative stress, depression appears to be a more hormonal related phenomena. Although chalcones aren't a hormone, let's not forget the potential correlation between the previous statement and the fact that they short of rev up hormone production and maintenance in plants.

When I began looking into chalcones a few years ago (I swore they were a sort of Spanish cuisine and I love Spanish food) I found something interesting about their anti attributes (meaning they fight against, the list is above). They are also known to be antimalarial, and Malaria is still a severe health problem in the world.

So Where Do All These Phytonutrients Come From?

So now you're fully aware of what these God given secondary metabolites can do for us. The biggest problem we're going to run into is where these nutritional powerhouses come from! That can be a daunting task, but seeing you've bought this book I'll let you know for free and save you the couple of hours it took for me to find them!

Let's start looking at carotenoids and find out where we can get them! I'll start with carotenoids, well because C comes before F in the alphabet, makes sense right? Without further delay and rambling here we go!

I'll make the list easy and just list everything in an A-Z manner and group everything together, sound good? Great, here we go!

Foods with Carotenoid Levels

Apricots

Asparagus (R)

Avocado (R)

Banana (R)

Beans (Green) (R)

Beets (Green) (R)

Broccoli (R)

Brussel Sprouts (R)

Cabbage (R)

Carrots (R)

Collard Greens (R)

Corn (Sweet & Yellow) (R)

Eggs (Whole & Fresh) (R)

Grapefruit (Pink & Red) (R)

Kale (R)

Lettuce (Cos & Romaine & Iceberg) (R)

Mango (R)

Melon (Cantaloupe) (R)

Nectarine (R)

Okra (R)

Oranges (R)

Orange Juice (Fresh if possible) (R)

Papaya (R)

Peach (R)

Peas (Green) (R)

Peppers (Green & Red) (R)

Pumpkin (R)

Spinach

Squash (Acorn, Crookneck, Straight, Summer, Winter, Zucchini) (R)

Sweet Potato (R)

Tangerine (R)

Tomato (Ripe) (R)

Watermelon (R)

This list is going to be a little different than the last, there's a great reason too! What's the reason it's more of a breakdown by group you may be asking? Well easy, there's a whole bunch more flavonoids than there is carotenoids. So I apologize for that, I should have warned you.

Dairy:

Milk

Herbs:

Basil (F)

Capers (Raw [Canned has some flavonoid makeup, however the difference is staggering])

Dill Weed (F)

Licorice Root

Oregano (F & Mexican)

Peppermint (F)

Rosemary (F)

Sage (F)

Spices:

Celery Seed (F)

Marjoram (D)

Parsley (F & D)

Saffron

Tarragon (F)

Thyme (F)

Fruit:

Acai (F)

Acai (White) (Frozen)

Acerola (R)

Apple (Cider, Juice, Raw, Fuji, Gala, Golden Delicious, Granny Smith, Red Delicious, Sauce [Canned])

Apricots (R)

Avocado (R)

Banana (Dwarf, Plantain) (R)

Bayberries

Bilberry (Soup) (R)

Blackberries (R)

Blueberries (Rabbiteye, Wild) (R)

Bog Whortleberries

Breadfruit

Cashew Apples

Cedar Bay Cherries

Cherries (Red, Sour, Sweet)

Chokeberries

Cloudberries

Coconuts (NON- Mature)

Cranberries (Bush, Sauce) (R)

Currants (European, Golden, Red, White) (R)

Dates

Elderberries (R)

Figs (R)

Goji Berry (R)

Gooseberries

Grape Juice

Grapefruit Juice (Pink, Red, White) (Unsweetened)

Frapes (Black, Concord, Green, Red, White)

Guava (Red & White flesh)

Juniper Berries (Both ripe and unripe are good)

Kiwi (Gold, Green, Red) (R)

Kumquats (R)

Lemon (R)

Limes (R)

Mangos (R)

Mulberries

Nectarines (White) (R)

Papaya (R)

Peaches (R)

Pears

Pineapple

Plum (Illawarra, Yellow, Black Diamond, Davidson's, Greengage, Purple,) (R)

Pomegranates

Raspberries (Black and Red)

Rhubarb Stalk (COOKED!)

Rhubarb (R)

Soursop

Strawberries (R)

Tangerines (R)

Watermelon (R)

Veggies:

Alfalfa

Artichokes

Arugula

Asparagus

Bay leaves (F)

Beans (butter, snap (green and yellow)

Beets (R)

Broccoli Raab (R)

Brussel Sprouts (R)

Cabbage (Chinese, Napa, Red, Savory) (R)

Carrots (R)

Cauliflower (R)

Celery Hearts (Green & White)

Celery (Chinese)

Chard (Swiss) (R)

Chicory Greens (R)

Chives

Collard Greens

Coriander leaves (R)

Eggplant (R)

Fennel (Bulb and Leaves)

Garlic

Ginger (R)

Kale (R)

Leeks (R)

Lettuce (Butterhead, Cos, Green Leaf, Red Leaf, Romaine)

Mustard Greens (R)

Okra (R)

Olive Leaves

Onions (Red, Spring, Sweet, Welsh, White, Young Green [TOPS ONLY!]) (R)

Parsley (F)

Peas (R)

Peppers (Ancho, Californian, Cayenne, Habanero, Hot Chili, Hot Yellow Wax, Jalapeno, Pimento, Serrano, Sweet [Green, Red, & Yellow])

Potatoes

Radish (R)

Soybeans

Spinach (R)

Squash

Sweet Potato(Leaves & Purple) (R)

Tomatoes (Cherry, Plum, Red, Yellow)

Watercress (R)

Nuts & Seeds:

Chia

Almonds

Brazilian Nuts

Cashews

Chestnuts

Coconut (water)

Hazelnuts

Macadamia

Pecan

Pistachios

Drinks:

Wine (Champagne, Cabernet Franc & Sauvignon, Sherry, Syrah, White)

Cocoa mix

Tea (Black, Fruit, Green, Oolong, White) (Brewed)

Legumes:

Beans (Black, Common, Kidney, Pinto, White)

Broadbeans

Carob (Fiber, Flour, Kibble,)

Chickpeas (R)

Cowpeas (R)

For the Sweet Tooth!

Baking Chocolate

Bee Pollen

Cacao Bean

Chocolate (Dark & Milk)

Grains:

Barley

Buckwheat (Bran and Flour)

Wheat

Phew, Did You Catch All That?

All of the chapters were placed into really short and bite sized pieces of information. Did you learn anything? If you did I have 2 really small favors to ask of you, actually I lied I have 3 favors and all of them are easy!

1. Implement the ideas you learned in this book (obviously after you tell your doctor what you're up to)
2. Leave a review on my Amazon listing (It'll help BIG TIME!)
3. Tell 5 friends or family members about this inexpensive book!

I appreciate it!

BY THE WAY! If you loved this book, you're going to want to check out these books too

Six Pack Fundamentals

Best Resistance Band

Naturally Improving Diabetes

How To Reverse Diabetes

Made in United States
Cleveland, OH
18 January 2025

13574119R00024